MW01595890

Ketogenic Bread Cookbook

Cookbook

Volume 2

By Anas Malla

Copyright 2017 - All rights reserved.

This document is geared towards providing exact and reliable information in regards to the topic and issue covered. The publication is sold with the idea that the publisher is not required to render accounting, officially permitted, or otherwise, qualified services. If advice is necessary, legal or professional, a practiced individual in the profession should be ordered.

- From a Declaration of Principles which was accepted and approved equally by a Committee of the American Bar Association and a Committee of Publishers and Associations.

In no way is it legal to reproduce, duplicate, or transmit any part of this document in either electronic means or in printed format. Recording of this publication is strictly prohibited and any storage of this document is not allowed unless with written permission from the publisher. All rights reserved.

The information provided herein is stated to be truthful and consistent, in that any liability, in terms of inattention or otherwise, by any usage or abuse of any policies, processes, or directions contained within is the solitary and utter responsibility of the recipient reader. Under no circumstances will any legal responsibility or blame be held against the publisher for any reparation, damages, or monetary loss due to the information herein, either directly or indirectly.

Respective authors own all copyrights not held by the publisher.

The information herein is offered for informational purposes solely, and is universal as so. The presentation of the information is without contract or any type of guarantee assurance.

The trademarks that are used are without any consent, and the publication of the trademark is without permission or backing by the trademark owner. All trademarks and brands within this book are for clarifying purposes only and are the owned by the owners themselves, not affiliated with this document.

Bonus!! FREE E-Book

This great book has a Bonus E-book called "10.5 Tips for Massive Success". You can download the book from my website.

I am honored and grateful to give you this free e-book, and I hope this will really help you to start your ketogenic diet, you can easy read it after downloading.

Thank you and enjoy reading.

If the links do not work, for whatever reason, you can simply visit my website:

Mastering-life.com/10successtipsbook

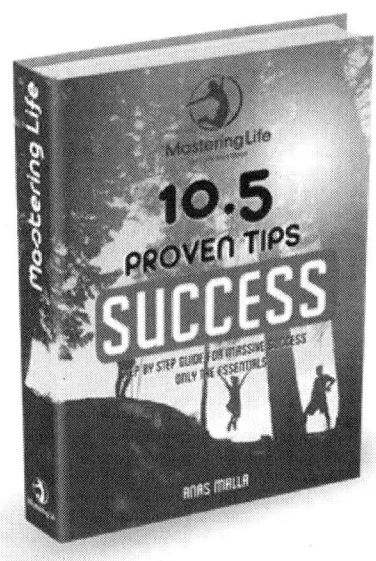

Table of Contents

Introduction

I want to thank you and congratulate you for downloading the book "**Ketogenic Bread Cookbook Vol. 2**"

This book contains 25 fantastic ketogenic bread recipes that perfectly fit with the ketogenic style of nutrition.

Tired of losing hours on the internet and in the bookstores looking for the best keto recipes? This book offers you an all-in-one solution – a bunch of tasty recipes sorted in various categories to suit all tastes.

The categories are:

- **Ketogenic bread recipes** – a total of 9 excellent recipes for all types of bread to make. Are you in the mood for a sweet snack or you would like the perfect loaf for your breakfast in the morning? I'm sure you will find what you are looking for in this book!
- **Ketogenic French toast** recipes – you don't have to give up on French toast when on keto diet, you just need someone to guide you to adapt it to your new way of nutrition
- **Ketogenic muffins recipes** – salty muffins perfect for your snack, spicy if you are looking for flavored options or sweet if you want to indulge your sweet tooth. They are all here!

- **Ketogenic waffles recipes** – tasty and delicious waffles made to fit with your diet
- **Ketogenic crackers and biscuits** – do you miss something to snack? Try these incredible cookies and biscuits' recipes and solve that problem!

As I said, a total of 25 recipes is at your disposal. I tested all of them myself, and I guarantee that you will include a bunch of them into your daily ketogenic nutrition. Everything is easier when you have a handy e-book like this one.

Thanks again for downloading this book, I hope you enjoy it!

Ketogenic Bread Recipes

Ultra-Quick Microwave Keto Bread
Serves 4

Ingredients

1 egg

1/3 cup almond flour

½ teaspoon baking powder

2 ½ tablespoons olive oil or butter

1/8 teaspoon salt

Directions

1. Grab a mug and grease it with oil or butter.
2. Use a small bowl to whisk an egg. After whisking it, add almond flour, baking powder, olive oil (butter), and salt. Use a fork to combine all the ingredients well.
3. Transfer the ingredients into the mug. Set microwave on HIGH and cook for 90 seconds. Allow it to cool down a bit before slicing.

Spicy Jalapeno Bread
Serves 4-6

Ingredients

6 big eggs

3 big jalapenos

4 ounces turkey bacon (or cheddar cheese)

½ cup ghee

½ cup coconut flour

¼ teaspoon baking soda

½ teaspoon salt

Directions

1. Turn your oven to 400F to preheat it. In the meantime, cut the 3 big jalapenos cut the big jalapenos into slices. Also, cut the turkey bacon (or cream cheese) into thick slices. Put jalapenos and bacon/cheese on a baking tray and roast for about 10 minutes. Make sure to flip them after 5 minutes.

2. Remove the seeds from the jalapenos and put them and bacon/cheese slices into a food processor or a blender. Pulse until you get a smooth consistency.

3. Use a big bowl to combine eggs, ghee, and ¼ cup of water. After you combine the ingredients, add coconut flour, baking soda, and salt and stir everything together. Finally, add the jalapeno-bacon mixture to the bowl.

4. Use a bit of ghee to grease a loaf pan and pour the batter into it. Bake for about 40 minutes at 375F. Allow it to cool down before serving.

Almond Keto Bread with Tartar Cream

Serves 10

Ingredients

6 big eggs

1 ½ cup almond flour

3 teaspoons baking powder

4 tablespoons butter

¼ teaspoon tartar cream

1/8 teaspoon salt

Directions

1. Turn your oven to 375F. Separate the eggs and add egg whites to one bowl and yolks to another. Add tartar cream to the bowl with egg whites and use an electric hand mixer to beat them until you get a soft peak form.

2. Use a food processor or a blender to process the yolks, almond flour, baking powder, butter, and salt. Combine the ingredients well.

3. Add a half of the egg whites mixture to the blender and continue pulsing until you mix the ingredients well. Next, insert the other half of the egg whites and process gently until the ingredients are thoroughly incorporated. At this point, you don't want to go too far in mixing the ingredients in order for the bread to keep its volume.

4. Add the batter to a loaf pan you should previously grease with butter or olive oil. Bake for about 30 minutes on 375F. Allow it to cool down before serving.

Ketogenic Psyllium Bread
Serves 10

Ingredients

10 ounces almond flour

3 ounces flaxseed meal

8 ounces egg whites

½ cup psyllium husk powder

3 ounces apple cider vinegar

1 ½ tablespoons baking powder

14 ounces boiling water

1 teaspoon salt

Directions

1. Turn your oven to 350F to preheat it. Use cooking spray to grease a loaf pan (rectangular is preferred).

2. Use a coffee grinder to grind the flaxseed meal to make it very fine. Add it to a big bowl and combine it with almond flour, psyllium powder, baking powder, and salt. You can use an electric hand mixer to combine all the ingredients well.

3. Grab a small bowl and add the egg whites and apple cider vinegar to it. Add the mixture to the large bowl with dry ingredients. Mix at high speed until the ingredients are incorporated. You shouldn't mix for more than 10 seconds in order for the bread to keep its volume.

4. Add the hot water evenly to the batter and continue mixing at high speed. Once again, 10 seconds should be enough, and you want to avoid overmixing.

5. Add the batter to the loaf pan and use your hands to shape it gently. Bake for about 90 minutes on 350F. Allow it to cool down before serving.

Banana Walnut Bread
Serves 8

Ingredients

3 big eggs

3 bananas

½ cup walnuts

2 cups almond flour

1 teaspoon baking soda

¼ cup olive oil

Directions

1. Turn your oven to 350F. Use cooking spray or olive oil to grease a loaf pan.
2. Cut the bananas into slices and add them to a medium bowl. Next, add the walnuts, eggs, olive oil, almond flour, and baking soda. Use an electric hand mixer to combine all the ingredients well.
3. Add the batter to the loaf pan. Bake for about 55 minutes or until the toothpick comes clean. Allow it to cool down before serving.

Chocolate Chip Cookies Bread
Serves 8

Ingredients

5 medium eggs

1 cup home-made macadamia butter

¼ cup coconut flour

2 tablespoons maple syrup

½ cup chocolate chips

2 teaspoons apple cider vinegar

1 tablespoon vanilla extract

½ teaspoon baking soda

½ teaspoon baking powder

Directions

1. We will make macadamia butter first. Put 2 cups of macadamia nuts in a bowl and cover it with water. Let the nuts absorb the water for about an hour. Rinse them well and then add them to a food processor or a blender. Process them until you get a creamy consistency. Be patient as this might take some time.

2. Turn your oven to 350F. Add 1 cup of macadamia butter you made to a bowl. You will probably make more than you need so that you can leave the rest in the fridge for future use.

3. Use a food processor or a blender and add eggs, baking powder, baking soda, coconut flour, vanilla extract, and apple cider vinegar to it. Process everything until the ingredients are smooth and well-combined. Add the chocolate chips to the mixture and use a spoon to stir them in. Add the butter to the mixture and combine until you mix the ingredients well.

4. Pour the batter into the loaf pan and even the top out. Bake for about 30 minutes at 350F. Allow it to cool down a bit before serving.

Coconut Zucchini Ketogenic Bread
Serves 12

Ingredients

¾ cup coconut flour

6 medium eggs

2 cups zucchini, shredded

½ cup coconut oil or melted butter

1 tablespoon fresh thyme

1 teaspoon baking soda

2 teaspoons apple cider vinegar

½ teaspoons garlic powder

½ teaspoon sea salt

Directions

1. Use a medium bowl to combine eggs, coconut oil or butter, zucchini, and apple cider vinegar. Mix until the ingredients are well combined.
2. Use another bowl and add coconut flour, garlic powder, thyme, baking powder, and salt. Combine everything until the ingredients are mixed.
3. Combine two bowls with the ingredients and mix everything well.
4. Use parchment paper to line a loaf pan and cooking spray to grease it. Pour the batter into the pan and sprinkle with more salt if you like it saltier.
5. Turn your oven to 350F and bake for around 60 minutes. Allow it to cool down before serving.

Banana Bread with Caramel Frosting
Serves 8

Ingredients

1/3 cup coconut flour

½ cup chia seed, ground

2 cups almond flour

1/3 cup whey protein powder, unflavored

¾ cup almond milk, unsweetened

¼ cup butter, melted

3 big eggs

1 teaspoon banana extract

1 tablespoon baking powder

½ teaspoon vanilla extract

½ cup Swerve or another sweetener of your choice

¼ teaspoon stevia extract

Frosting:

¼ cup Swerve or another sweetener of your choice, powdered

4 ounces cream cheese

1 teaspoon caramel flavor

6 tablespoons whipping cream

Directions

1. Turn your oven to 325F. Use olive oil or butter to grease a loaf pan.
2. Grab a bowl and add ground chia seed and water. You can grind chia seeds in a coffee grinder. Let the mixture sit for about 30 minutes in order for the seeds to absorb the water. Your goal is to get a consistency of mashed bananas. If needed, add more water.
3. Grab a big bowl and add coconut flour, almond flour, Swerve or another sweetener, whey protein powder, salt, and baking powder. Combine the ingredients well.
4. Add almond milk, melted butter, vanilla extract, banana extract, stevia extract, eggs, and ground chia mixture. Stir the ingredients until you thoroughly combine them.
5. Transfer the mixture to the loaf pan and even out the top. Bake for around 70 minutes at 325F or until the top becomes golden brown.
6. Make the frosting by combining powdered sweetener and softened cream cheese in a big bowl. Next, add caramel flavor and whipping cream and continue beating until you combine the ingredients well. Spread the frosting over the bread and allow it to cool down before serving.

Cheesy Rosemary Bread
Serves 8

Ingredients

2 eggs

¾ cup plain yogurt

½ cup Parmesan cheese

1 cup cheddar cheese

1 head of cauliflower

1 teaspoon oregano

1 teaspoon basil

1 tablespoon rosemary

½ teaspoon thyme

Salt and pepper to taste

Directions

1. Turn your oven to 400F to preheat it. Use a food processor to grate the cauliflower head.
2. Grab a big bowl and add eggs, yogurt, Parmesan cheese, cheddar cheese, oregano, basil, thyme, rosemary, and cauliflower. Adjust the seasoning with salt and pepper and combine all the ingredients well.
3. Use parchment paper to line baking sheet and grease it with a cooking spray. Spread the batter evenly over the baking sheet. Bake for about 45 minutes at 400F. During the final 10 minutes of baking, you can sprinkle cheddar cheese over the bread to make it even tastier.

Get FREE Access To
"30 Days Ketogenic Plan"

Printable – Table

Go to: http://bit.ly/2pVjqJ7

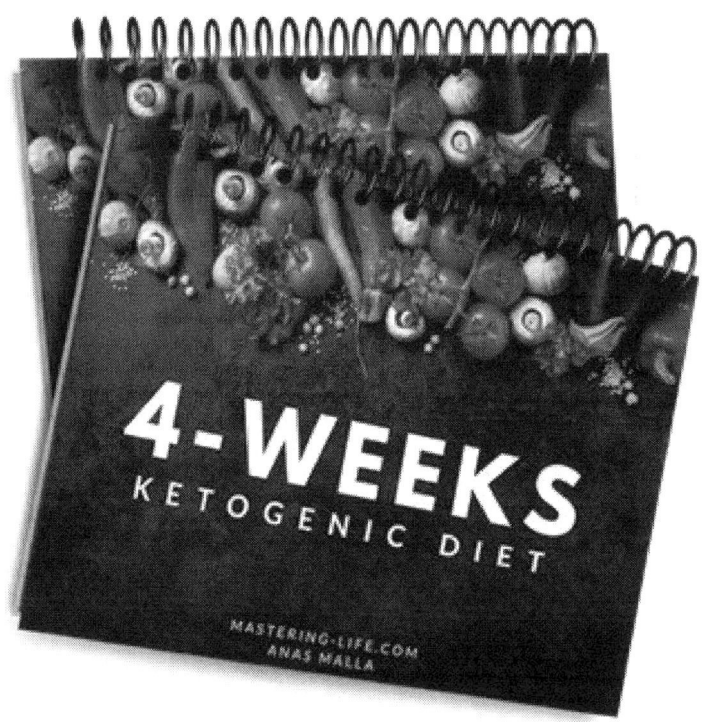

Ketogenic French Toast Recipes

Macadamia French Toast
Serves 2

Ingredients

1 big egg

1 ounce macadamia nuts

½ tablespoon butter

2 teaspoon coconut flour

½ teaspoon cinnamon

3 tablespoons maple syrup

¼ teaspoon baking powder

1 pinch ground nutmeg

1 teaspoon vanilla extract

Directions

1. You will need a microwave-safe mug or a bowl (even a ramekin will do). Add 1 ounce of macadamia nuts to a blender or a food processor and grind them for a bit. You don't want to over-process it to avoid making macadamia butter.
2. Add egg, softened butter, maple syrup, macadamia nuts, coconut flour, baking powder, vanilla extract, ground nutmeg, and cinnamon to the bowl or a mug you chose. Combine all the ingredients well to make a smooth mixture.
3. Insert the bowl into the microwave and cook for 2 to 3 minutes. It depends on the strength of your device, and you will have to figure out the required time yourself. The goal is to make a spongy and soft batter.
4. Remove from the mug and cut the dough in half. Put it in the toaster of a frying pan to brown on both sides. You can sprinkle maple syrup, cinnamon, or more butter right before serving.

Ricotta Cheese French Toast
Serves 1

Ingredients

¼ cup almond flour

¼ cup Stevia or another sweetener of your choice

1 tablespoon coconut flour

4 eggs

¾ cup ricotta cheese

½ teaspoon xanthan gum

1 tablespoon butter

1 teaspoon cinnamon

½ teaspoon salt

Directions

1. Turn your oven to 350F. Separate the eggs and put whites and yolks into different bowls. Use an electric hand mixer to whisk the egg whites until you get a stiff peak form. Put them into the refrigerator to cool down.

2. Add Stevia or sweetener of your choice and salt to the yolks. Mix them until you lighten the yolks. Add xanthan gum and ricotta cheese. Vigorously whisk the ingredients to avoid xanthan to clump.

3. Add coconut flour and almond flour and mix until the ingredients are well combined. You should get a thick batter consistency.

4. Remove the egg whites from the refrigerator and add a half of it to the yolk mixture. Use a rubber spatula to mix the ingredients. Next, add the remaining half of the batter and fold carefully. Cut the spatula into the center of the bowl and make sure to fold from the bottom to the top, turning the bowl four times in the process. Your goal is to keep folding until you don't see any egg whites left.

5. Use a nonstick skillet to melt butter over low temperature. Remove any excess butter and transfer the batter to the pan. Fry it on low heat for about a minute.

6. Transfer the batter to the oven and bake at 350F until the top starts to brown and the mixture sets.

Ketogenic Muffins Recipes

Egg Muffins
Serves 6

Ingredients

6 eggs

6 cheddar cheese small slices

1 handful spinach

4 cherry tomatoes

3 spring onions

1 red bell pepper

½ teaspoon salt

Directions

1. Turn your oven to 390F to preheat it. Use a big mixing bowl and add cherry tomatoes, onions, and red bell pepper to it. Don't forget to wash the veggies fist.
2. Chop the spinach and add it to the bowl. Next, add eggs and salt (you can adjust the seasoning to taste). Combine all the ingredients well.
3. Use cooking spray or olive oil to grease the muffin cups (you will need 6 of them). Transfer the batter into the muffin tins and make sure to distribute it evenly across all of them.
4. Put one small slice of cheddar cheese over each of the muffins. Bake for 18 minutes at 390F or until the top of the cupcakes get firm to the touch.

Macadamia Muffins
Serves 12

Ingredients

2 cups macadamia nuts, unsalted

½ cup almond flour

2/3 cup coconut, shredded, toasted

¼ cup Stevia or sweetener of your choice

2 tablespoons whey protein powder, unflavored

6 ounces softened cream cheese

¼ cup almond milk, unsweetened

2 eggs

½ teaspoon baking soda

½ cup macadamia nuts, chopped

2 teaspoons baking powder

10 drops stevia extract

2 teaspoons lime zest

½ teaspoon salt

¼ cup coconut oil, melted

Topping:

1/3 cup powdered sweetener of your choice

2 tablespoons lime juice

Directions

1. Turn your oven to 325F to preheat it. Use parchment paper to line the muffin cups (you will need 12 of them).

2. Use a food processor or a blender and add macadamia nuts to it. Process them until you make them finely ground (it shouldn't take long). Be careful not to make macadamia butter – you only want it ground!

3. Move the nuts to a bowl and add almond flour, shredded coconut, Stevia or sweetener of your choice, whey protein powder, baking powder, baking soda, lime zest, and salt. Whisk the ingredients until you combine them well.

4. Grab another bowl and lightly beat the eggs. Add the macadamia mixture to it and continue beating until you combine the ingredients well. Add almond milk, coconut oil, and stevia extract and continue mixing until you completely combine all the ingredients. Add the chopped macadamia nuts and stir them in.

5. Transfer the batter to the muffin tins and make sure to distribute it equally across the cups. Bake for 25 minutes at 325F. Allow it to cool down a bit.

6. Prepare the topping by combining powdered sweetener of your choice and lime juice in a bowl. You should get a smooth mixture that you can drizzle over the muffins once they cool down.

Spicy Pumpkin Muffins
Serves 12

Ingredients

6 big eggs

1 cup coconut, shredded

2 cups almond flour

3/4 cup canned pumpkin puree, unsweetened

1/3 cup coconut flour

3/4 cup canned coconut milk

1/3 cup pumpkin kernels, chopped

1/3 cup sunflower seeds, chopped

1/2 cup Stevia or sweetener of your choice

2 tablespoons psyllium husk powder

1 tablespoon vinegar

1/2 teaspoon baking soda

1 teaspoon baking powder

1/2 teaspoon stevia glycerite

1/2 teaspoon mace, ground

1/4 teaspoon ginger, ground

1/4 teaspoon cinnamon, ground

1/2 teaspoon maple extract

1/2 teaspoon salt

Directions

1. Turn your oven to 350F to preheat it. Use cooking spray to grease muffin tins (you will need 12 of them).
2. Use a food processor or a blender to pulse the shredded coconut and nuts.
3. Grab a big mixing bowl and add ground coconut-nut mixture to it. Add almond flour, coconut flour, psyllium husk powder, baking powder, baking soda, Stevia, ground mace, ground cinnamon, ground ginger, and salt. Combine everything until you mix the ingredients well.
4. Use another bowl to mix 6 big eggs, pumpkin puree, coconut milk, vinegar, stevia glycerite, and maple extract. Combine everything well. Once you mix all the ingredients thoroughly, add them to the big bowl with nut mixture in it. Combine everything once again until all the ingredients are incorporated. Allow it to sit for about 7-8 minutes.
5. Transfer the batter to the muffin cups. Make sure to divide it equally between the 12 tins. Bake for 8 minutes at 400F and then reduce the heat to 350F and continue baking for another 30 minutes. It depends on the oven, but the muffins are done once the toothpick comes out clean, and they become golden brown.

Carrot Zucchini Muffins
Serves 12

Ingredients

3 medium eggs

6 tablespoons coconut flour

1 ½ teaspoon baking powder

1/3 cup Stevia or sweetener of your choice

1 tablespoon golden flax meal

½ cup zucchini, grated

1/3 cup carrot, grated

¼ cup almond milk, unsweetened

¼ teaspoon baking soda

1 teaspoon cinnamon

½ teaspoon apple cider vinegar

1 teaspoon vanilla extract

2 tablespoon butter or olive oil

Topping:

1 teaspoon vanilla extract

1 teaspoon lemon juice

4 ounces cream cheese

½ teaspoon liquid stevia

Directions

1. Turn your oven to 350F to preheat it. Use a big bowl and add coconut flour, Stevia or sweetener of your choice, cinnamon, baking soda, baking powder, and golden flax meal to it. Combine the ingredients until they are well mixed and allow them to sit for a bit.

2. Grab a different bowl and add the eggs, grated zucchini, grated carrot, almond milk, vanilla extract, apple cider vinegar, and butter or olive oil. Combine all the ingredients until they are well mixed.

3. Transfer the batter to the muffin tins and divide it equally across 12 cups. Bake for about 30 minutes at 350F or until the muffins get golden brown color (the toothpick should come out clean). Allow them to cool down completely.

4. In the meantime, make the frosting by combining cream cheese, lemon juice, vanilla extract, and liquid stevia in a bowl. Use an electric hand mixer to combine all the ingredients until you get a creamy consistency. Put the topping over the muffins once they cool down and serve.

Cranberry Almond Muffins
Serves 12

Ingredients

6 big eggs

½ cup + 2 tablespoons Swerve or sweetener of your choice

½ cup coconut flour

2 cups almond flour

1 tablespoon apple cider vinegar

½ teaspoon baking soda

½ teaspoon stevia glycerite

2 teaspoons baking powder

1 ½ cups cranberries, fresh, chopped

½ cup coconut milk

2 tablespoons psyllium husk powder

½ teaspoon almond extract

1 teaspoon vanilla extract

¼ cup almonds, sliced

1 tablespoon melted butter

½ teaspoon salt

Directions

1. Turn your oven to 350F to preheat it. Use cooking spray to grease the muffin tins (you will need 12 of them). Use a food processor to chop the fresh cranberries and allow them to sit for a bit.

2. Use a bowl and add almond flour, coconut flour, ½ cup of Swerve, baking powder, baking soda, and salt. Combine everything until there are no lumps in the batter. Set aside 1/3 of the dough because you will need it later.

3. Add the psyllium husk powder to the remaining muffin batter and stir it in. Once you stir, top the mixture with chopped cranberries.

4. Grab another bowl and add eggs, apple cider vinegar, almond extract, vanilla extract, and stevia glycerite. Use an electric hand mixer or a fork to combine all the ingredients well.

5. Add the egg mixture to the chopped cranberries mixture. Mix all the ingredients until they are well combined. Allow the batter to sit for about 7-8 minutes.

6. Use a small bowl and combine the 1/3 of the muffin mixture you saved with sliced almonds, 2 tablespoons of Swerve, and 1 tablespoon of melted butter. Use a fork or even your fingers to mix the ingredients for a bit.

7. Divide the batter (the one with eggs and cranberries) equally across 12 of the muffin tins you previously greased. Place the sliced almonds mixture on top of the muffins.
8. Bake for about 6 minutes at 400F and then reduce the heat to 350F and bake for additional 20 minutes. It depends on the oven, but the muffins are done once the toothpick comes out clean, and they become golden brown.

Mocha Chocolate Chunks Muffins
Serves 12

Ingredients

1 ½ cup almond flour

¼ cup cocoa, unsweetened

1 cup dark chocolate bar, chopped

½ cup flax seed meal

1 tablespoon instant coffee granules

½ cup melted butter

2 teaspoons baking powder

3 eggs

½ cup of Swerve or sweetener of your choice

Directions

1. Turn your oven to 350F to preheat it. Use cooking spray to grease the muffin cups (you will need 12 of them).
2. Boil a ¼ cup of water and add the coffee granules to it. Once they dissolve, set them aside to cool down for a bit.
3. Use a medium bowl to mix flax seed meal, almond flour, baking powder, and cocoa.
4. Once they are combined, add eggs, melted butter, sweetener of your choice, and coffee. Continue stirring until you combine all the ingredients.
5. Chop the chocolate bar and add it to the mixture. Stir the batter to distribute the chocolate evenly all over it.
6. Transfer the batter into the muffin tins. Make sure to divide the dough across all 12 muffin cups proportionally. Bake for 14 minutes at 350F. Allow them to cool down before serving.

Maple Pecan Muffins
Serves 12

Ingredients

½ cup Almond Flour

¼ cup Flaxseed

1/3 cup pecan halves

1 large egg

1 tablespoon vanilla extract

1 tablespoon maple extract

¼ cup coconut oil

1/8 cup erythritol

1/8 tablespoon stevia (liquid)

¼ tablespoon baking soda

¼ tablespoon apple cider vinegar

Directions

1. Turn your oven to 325F to preheat it. Put pecan halves into a food processor or a blender to coarsely chop them.
2. Grab a bowl and add the egg, maple extract, vanilla extract, stevia, apple cider vinegar, and coconut oil.
3. Use a different bowl to mix 2/3 of pecan halves with almond flour, flaxseed, baking soda, and erythritol. Make sure to combine the ingredients well.
4. Add the pecan mixture to the egg mixture and combine them until you make a dough form.
5. Transfer the batter into muffin molds and make sure to divide them equally between the tins (you will need 12 of them). Sprinkle the top with the remaining pecans.
6. Bake for 30 minutes at 325F. Allow the muffins to cool down before serving.

Get FREE Access To

"11 Ketogenic Food Lists"

Go to: http://bit.ly/2pa7IrX

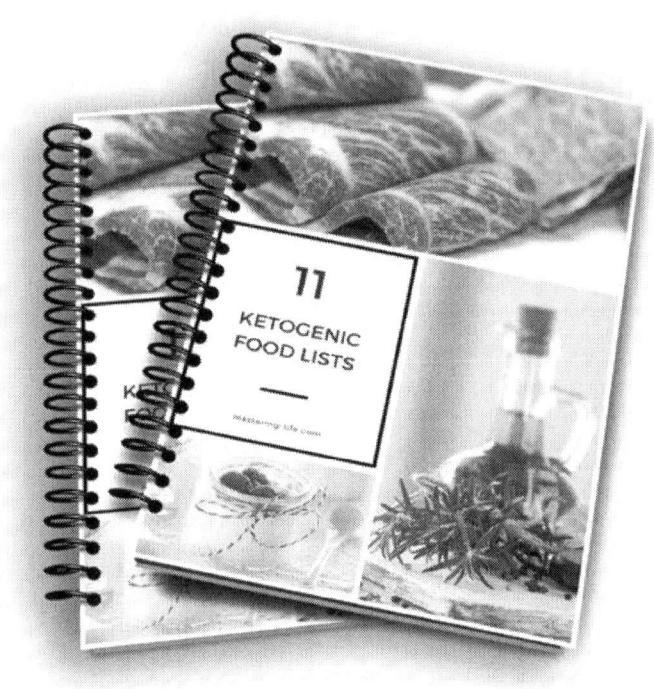

Ketogenic Waffles Recipes

Sweet Potato Waffles
Serves 4

Ingredients

1 egg

1 cup sweet potatoes, mashed

1 teaspoon garlic

¼ cup coconut flour

¼ cup olive oil

Salt to taste

Directions

1. Turn on your waffle maker to preheat it. Don't forget to grease it well to prevent the batter from sticking.
2. Add sweet potatoes, egg, coconut flour, garlic, and salt to taste to a food processor or a blender. Process all ingredients.
3. Transfer the batter onto griddles, making sure that you cover each section with the equal amount of batter. Repeat until you have batter remaining.

Cinnamon Soy Flour Waffles
Serves 8

Ingredients

3 eggs

¾ cup buttermilk

1 cup soy flour

1 tablespoon baking powder

6 tablespoons Swerve or sweetener of your choice

1/3 cup melted butter

½ teaspoon baking soda

1 teaspoon vanilla extract

2 tablespoons ground cinnamon

Directions

1. Turn your waffle iron on to preheat it. Use a mixing bowl and add soy flour, baking soda, baking powder, ground cinnamon, and Swerve or sweetener of your choice to it. Combine all the ingredients well.
2. Add melted butter, eggs, buttermilk, and vanilla extract and mix all the ingredients until you combine them well.
3. Add about a ½ cup of cold water to the batter. Make sure to add it gradually. You want to make your batter a bit thick, so you don't have to use all water if you achieved this with lesser quantity.
4. Transfer the dough to your preheated waffle iron. You should use around 1/3 cup of batter each time. Once the waffle browns a bit on both sides, remove it from the pan. Repeat the process until you have no more batter remaining.

Sage and Cheddar Waffles
Serves 6

Ingredients

2/3 cup coconut flour

1 cup canned coconut milk

1/2 cup cheddar cheese

1 ½ tablespoon melted coconut oil

1 whole egg

1/2 tablespoon dried ground sage

1/2 tablespoon garlic powder

1 ½ tablespoons baking powder

1/4 tablespoon of salt

Directions

1. Turn your waffle iron to preheat it. Grab a bowl and add the coconut flour, baking powder, and all the seasonings to it. Combine the ingredients well.
2. Add the wet ingredients and combine everything to make a batter form.
3. Finally, add the shredded cream cheese to the batter and combine everything well.
4. Transfer the batter to the waffle iron and make the waffles. Allow them to cool down a bit before serving.

Get FREE Access To

"Pros & Cons of The Ketogenic Diet"

Go to: http://bit.ly/2rrnEM1

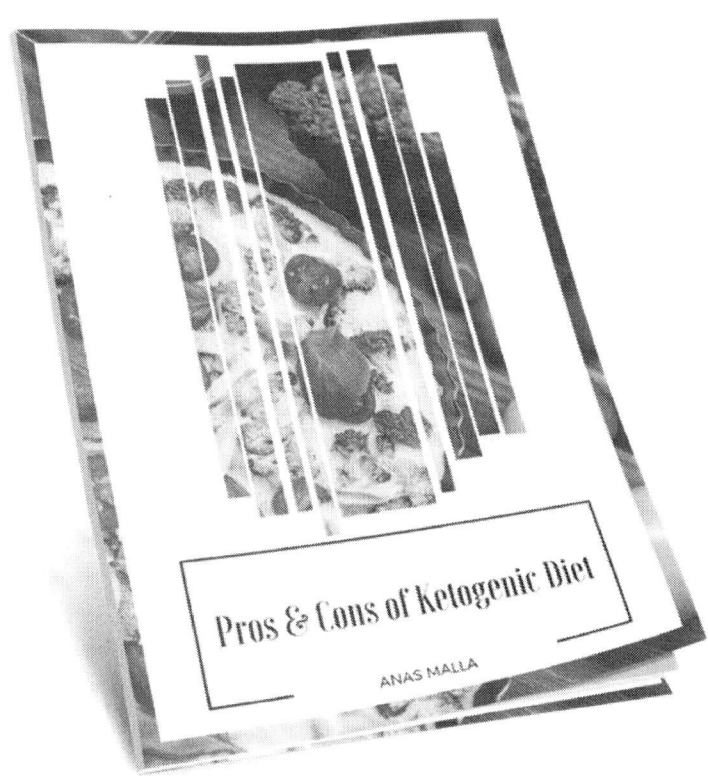

Ketogenic Biscuits and Crackers

Coconut Flour Biscuits
Serves 8

Ingredients

4 big eggs

½ cup coconut flour

½ teaspoon baking powder

2 tablespoons maple syrup

5 tablespoons of melted butter (or coconut oil)

Salt to taste

Directions

1. Turn your oven to 400F to preheat it. Grab a bowl and add coconut flour, eggs, maple syrup, baking powder, melted butter (or coconut oil), and salt to taste. Use an electric hand mixer to combine all the ingredients. Alternatively, you can even use a blender to process them.
2. Once the ingredients are well incorporated, for 8 small patties. Use a spoon to flatten them. You want each to remind you of biscuits, so they should have about 1-2 inch thickness.
3. Bake for 15 minutes at 400F. It depends on the oven, but the biscuits are done once they begin to brown a bit.

Parmesan Garlic Biscuits
Serves 24

Ingredients

6 eggs

¾ cup Parmesan cheese, grated

1 cup almond flour

2 teaspoons baking powder

1/3 cup coconut flour

1 tablespoon parsley, dried

6 garlic cloves, minced

1/3 cup melted butter (or coconut oil)

Directions

1. Turn your oven to 350F to preheat it. Use parchment paper to line a baking sheet.
2. Use a big bowl and add almond flour, coconut flour, grated parmesan cheese, baking powder, and parsley to it. Combine the ingredients well.
3. Add eggs and melted butter (or coconut oil) to the mix and stir everything until you combine the ingredients. Allow it to sit for about 5 minutes for the batter to thicken.
4. Use a spoon to transfer the batter to the baking sheet. In the process, make biscuits shapes. You need about one tablespoonful to make one cookie. You can also use a cookie scooper. If you want, you can sprinkle with more Parmesan cheese.
5. Bake for 20 minutes at 350F. It depends on the oven, but the cookies are done once they reach golden color and become firm to the touch. Allow them to cool down before serving.

Ketogenic Cheese Crackers
Serves 6

Ingredients

1 egg

1 cup almond flour

2 cups Parmesan cheese

2 ounces cream cheese

1 teaspoon rosemary

½ teaspoon salt

Directions

1. Use a microwave-safe bowl and add almond flour, cream cheese, and Parmesan cheese to it. Combine the ingredients and put them in the microwave. Cook for 60 seconds using the HIGH settings. Your goal is to melt the cheese partially. Make sure to stir the mixture as soon as you take it out of the microwave.

2. Allow the mixture to sit for a bit and then add the egg, rosemary, and salt. Combine all the ingredients until you mix them well. If the cheese gets too hard, you can put it in the microwave for 10 more seconds to soften it.

3. Use parchment paper to line a baking sheet. Transfer a large ball of dough on the sheet and put another piece of the parchment paper over it (it should be the same size). Next, spread the batter to make a thin layer.

4. You can use a pizza cutter or a knife to make square crackers from the dough. Bake for 12 minutes at 450F, making sure to flip once after 6 minutes. Allow them to cool down a bit before serving.

Almond Sesame Crackers
Serves 4

Ingredients

1 cup almond flour

1 big egg

¼ teaspoon baking soda

3 tablespoons sesame seeds

Salt and pepper

Directions

1. Turn your oven to 350F to preheat it. Use parchment paper to line up a baking sheet.
2. Grab a bowl and add almond flour, baking soda, sesame seeds, and salt and pepper to taste. Combine all the ingredients well.
3. Add the egg and combine the ingredients again to make a batter. Next, cut the dough into two halves.
4. Put parchment paper on a working area and use cooking spray to grease it. Place the batter in the center and make a form a ball. Next, put another piece of parchment paper over it (don't forget to spray it, too).
5. Make a large rectangle out of the batter. Take off the top parchment paper and slice the dough into crackers by using a knife or a pizza cutter. You can add additional salt and pepper if you want to.
6. Put the dough on the baking sheet and bake for about 20 minutes. Allow them to cool down before serving. If you can't bake the entire batter at once, you can bake one-half at a time.

Conclusion

Thank you again for downloading this book!

I hope you've had fun reading this book and preparing some of the amazing ketogenic recipes listed here.

My goal was to provide you various recipes that will suit different tastes. I'm sure that each of you managed to find a lot of tasty meals that you will prepare on a regular basis during your ketogenic style of nutrition.

Finally, if you enjoyed this book, then I'd like to ask you for a favor, would you be kind enough to leave a review for this book on Amazon? It'd be greatly appreciated.

Visit the link below to leave a review:
https://www.amazon.com/review/create-review

For more information, please check out my blog at: **Mastering-life.com**

Thank you and good luck!

Preview Of
"Ketogenic Fat Bombs" Book
Introduction

I want to thank you and congratulate you for downloading the book "**Ketogenic Fat Bombs, Sweets, and Snacks**"!

This book contains recipes for fat bombs, sweets, and snacks that perfectly fit your ketogenic diet plan.

If you didn't know, the ketogenic diet is one of the quickest and safest way to get your weight in order. It was never that easy to lose all those extra pounds like with the ketogenic diet.

However, some of the people have problems with finding enough different recipes for their nutrition plan. They say that it is especially tricky with fat bombs. Well, not anymore!

This book offers you more than 60 recipes and covers:

- **Ketogenic fat bombs** – sweet and salty recipes perfect for everyone
- **Ketogenic sweets** – dessert recipes ideal for indulging your sweet tooth
- **Ketogenic snacks** – if you are looking for a boost of energy of you don't feel quite full after a meal

And much more!

As someone who is on the ketogenic diet, I tried to select the most tasteful recipes that are at the same time easy to prepare. If you are looking for simple fat bombs, sweets and snacks recipes for keto diet, then you can find all that here.

Thanks again for downloading this book, I hope you enjoy it!

Chapter 1 – Fat Bombs

What Are Ketogenic Fat Bombs?

A lot of people are paranoid when it comes to eating fat. Although it has been public enemy number one for a long time, research has confirmed that fats can be extremely healthy. The only condition you need to fulfill is to choose the right type of fats. According to scientific reports, saturated fats that we can find in butter, coconut oil, cream cheese and even heavy cream influence our levels of good cholesterol. That improves the chances of avoiding and fighting heart disease, decreases our blood pressure, enhances our overall healthy and, last but not least, gets our weight in order.

A fat bomb is most similar to an energy bar or, more precisely, an energy ball. However, those energy bars that you can get in your local store are usually not as close to the fat content you should aim for. Each of the fat bomb recipes we offer has more than 75% of fat content and, more often than not, the amount of fat is over 85%. Unlike energy bars, fat bombs don't have sugar-heavy or carb-rich ingredients. Instead, they are just focused on ingredients that add a lot of fat and almost no carbs, like coconut oil, cream or peanut butter.

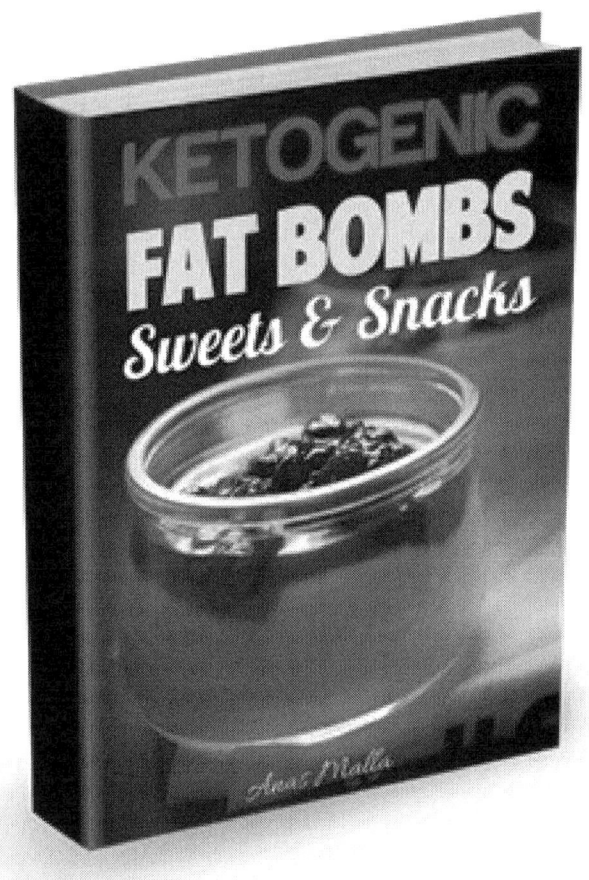

If you are wondering when you can eat these fat bombs, the answer is – any time you want! They can be a great and quick breakfast, an excellent mid-afternoon snack or maybe even dinner, as long as they fit into your daily nutrition plan.

Fat bombs usually have ingredients from these three categories:

- **Healthy fats** – coconut butter, almond butter, peanut butter, cocoa butter, cream cheese, ghee...
- **Low-carb flavoring** – sugar-free dark chocolate, cocoa powder, vanilla extract, spices, salt...
- **Texture ingredients** – nuts, shredded coconuts, seeds...

Why Do You Need Ketogenic Fat Bombs?

As I mentioned, there are some fats that are bad, and these are called trans fats. On the other hand, there are "good fat's" that you should be eating to help our organism dissolve different vitamins, including vitamin A, D, E, and K. Fat bombs also help reduce our bad cholesterol levels (LDL) and improve the amount of good cholesterol (HDL).

Those of you who are aiming to get rid of extra pounds will surely be delighted to hear that fat bombs can help us get our weight in order. Each of these recipes perfectly fits into ketogenic diet plans. Naturally, you will need to track your portion sizes or, in other words, you can't eat too many of these fat bombs.

Now that we are familiar with what fat bombs are let's move on to the recipes. I also included several recipes that are rich in healthy fats and also fit perfectly with your ketogenic diet.

Go to this link to check out the rest of the "**Ketogenic Fat Bombs**" book:

http://amzn.to/2qDgS4U

Check Out My Other Books

Below you'll find some of my other popular books that are popular on Amazon and Kindle as well. Simply click on the links below to check them out.

Alternatively, you can visit my "Author Page" on Amazon to see other work done by me:

Anas Malla: http://amzn.to/2nzCevB

- **Ketogenic Diet**
  http://amzn.to/2ps3ePm

- **Ketogenic Bread Cookbook V.1**
  http://amzn.to/2m8hixm

- **Instant Pot Ketogenic Cookbook V.1**
  http://amzn.to/2o4oCfP

- **Instant Pot Ketogenic Cookbook V.2**
  http://amzn.to/2o4oCfP

- **Ketogenic Fat Bombs**
  http://amzn.to/2qDgS4U

- **Minimalist Living**
  http://amzn.to/2phTu8M

- **Conversation Tactics**
  http://amzn.to/2oj23Qg

If the links do not work, for whatever reason, you can simply search for these titles on the Amazon website to find them.

49422512R00041

Made in the USA
Middletown, DE
16 October 2017